Healing Self-Care Primer

How To create a DIY Self-Care Health & Healing Program.

Author Edward G. Palmer sheds light on self-care, alternative health, and DIY healing strategies.

Healing Self-Care Primer

Healing Self-Care Primer

*How To Create a Self-Care
Health & Healing Program.*

Edward G. Palmer

Healing Self-Care Primer: How To Create A Self-Care Health & Healing Program.

Publisher:

JVED Publishing
13570 Grove Drive #361
Maple Grove MN 55311
http://www.jvedpublishing.org

Print Edition

ISBN 9798868386831
All Rights Reserved

Disclaimer: This book is the sole opinion of the author based on his research, knowledge, and understanding. It is not intended to provide medical advice and is solely for educational purposes. Anyone in need of medical assistance should seek the appropriate expertise within the medical industry.

*Dedicated to everyone who takes responsibility
for their own health and healing!*

Table Of Contents

A special thanks to my wife Becky for her creative thoughts, editorial inputs, and encouragement.

CHAPTER ONE
Introducing Healing Self-Care Author

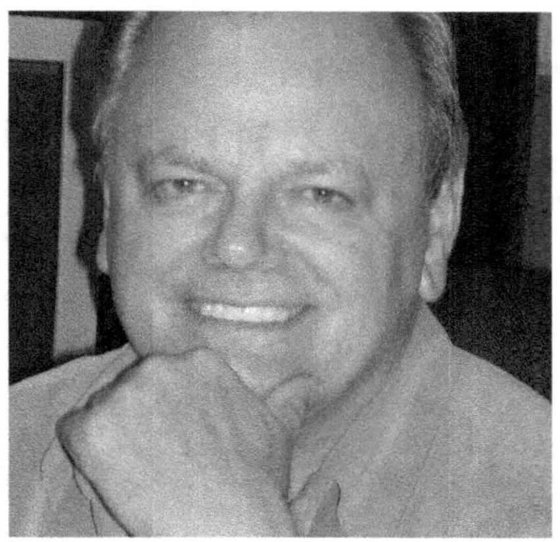

Edward G. Palmer

Hello, and thank you for reading this short eBook on "Healing Self-Care: A DIY Primer." I am author Edward G. Palmer. For 50 years, I have practiced "Healing Self-Care." I believe that any vocation or calling practiced for 50 years will make you somewhat of an expert in that area of study. Therefore, it's common for people to seek out my thoughts on Healing Self-Care. My purpose in writing is to shed light on healing self-care, alternative healing strategies, and spiritual wisdom. It is my hope that my writings will expose you to cost-effective healing self-care and low-cost alternative healing strategies. I also write to teach spiritual wisdom for healing our bodies and souls that is also not widely known or understood.

A detailed author's website is at http://www.edwardgpalmer.com. There, you will find a complete bio and other information, including my health and healing blog. At this site, you will find two books on health and healing. Having lost my first wife to pancreatic cancer after 39 years of marriage and being a spiritual man, I wrote a small book about what the Bible actually says about healing[1]. I now have over 50 years of experience with alternative healing strategies.

The second health and healing book was written while I was recovering from a stroke. It left me seeing double images, and my eyesight was severely impaired at age 76. Yes, I am healed.

I explained the approach to my healing in this book and how family, friends, and doctors became unglued when I refused to get an MRI to check for brain tumors. You'll find a more detailed DIY approach to health and healing in my book "The Doctor's Death Diagnosis[2]."

These two health and healing books, along with my blog on health and healing, constitute my effort to help people understand they have other options for healing than going to the doctor or hospital. I refer to these as cost-effective alternative health and healing strategies. Yes, there is a better way to take care of your health and healing than becoming financially drained by an out-of-control medical insurance industry.

Is It Health Care - Or A Health Protection Racket?

Suppose you've come to believe that standardized medical care and medical insurance with high deductibles are bankrupting you and your family. In that case, you'll need both of my books to fully understand that a different approach to health and healing exists. You'll find low-cost eBooks for both books to help guide you into another health and healing strategy. One focused on actually improving health instead of focusing on excessive medical system costs for just health care protection.

Are you facing $12,000 to $16,000 or more in annual medical premiums and $8,000 to $12,000 in deductible costs? That means you must meet $20,000-28,000 in out-of-pocket expenses before you realize a single dime in actual healthcare payouts. I've heard these types of numbers from several people. They're shocking, and health care, as it presently exists in the USA, is rapidly becoming unaffordable for many families.

The days of employers taking care of medical costs for their employees are long gone. Most employees are now facing high premiums along with high deductibles. I don't blame employers. It is an out-of-control medical healthcare system. There are too many lawsuits and unnecessary tests and surgeries, adding to the overall cost of medical care.

Recent government dole-outs imply that it may be more cost-effective to not work and go on government assistance if you have serious medical issues. Some poor people might even consider crime and imprisonment for health care. When healthcare policies in society are better for prison inmates than they are for working people--something has gone awry with the healthcare system.

What Exactly Is Health Care?

Are you paying for health care protection instead of actual and natural health care? Does your health care or medical plan coverage pay for any incurred medical or dental costs before your deductible is reached? Depending on how much you can pay each month, your plan may not pay much of anything, or it may cover all of your medical costs.

In one instance, you are paying medical costs that might threaten you with bankruptcy. In the other case, you have no out-of-pocket expenses. Instead, you have a hefty monthly payment to some insurance company. How much can you afford each month, and what happens if you get sick while out of the plan's coverage network?

CHAPTER TWO
Healthcare Complaints

Here is a list of several common healthcare complaints in the USA concerning doctors, hospitals, and medical insurance companies. These complaints vary depending on individual experiences and circumstances, but some of the most common grievances include:

1. **Billing and Insurance Issues:** This includes surprise medical bills, incorrect billing, denial of claims, lack of transparency in pricing, and difficulty in understanding insurance coverage or navigating the claims process.

   Note: My current wife was once charged over $500 for a five-minute session with an ear doctor who only offered a toxic drug to consume. My wife rejected the drug advice and took the necessary 3-4 months to get over the ear problem. Yes, many of our health problems will resolve naturally over a few weeks or months without any doctor visit. Yet it cost my family $500 for *bad advice and ineffective treatment.*

2. **Lack of Access and Long Wait Times:** Many patients complain about difficulties getting timely doctor appointments, long wait times in hospitals or emergency departments, and limited access to specialized care in certain areas.

3. **Communication and Bedside Manner:** Patients often express dissatisfaction with doctors' lack of communication, rushed appointments, inadequate explanations of medical conditions and treatment options, and a perceived lack of empathy or bedside manner.

4. **Medical Errors and Misdiagnosis:** Complaints regarding medical errors, misdiagnosis, delayed diagnosis, and medication errors, which can result in harm, extended hospital stays, or unnecessary treatments.

5. **Inadequate Time with Doctors:** Some patients feel that doctors do not spend enough time with them during appointments, leading to rushed consultations and limited opportunities for asking questions or addressing concerns.

Note: A recent medical doctor's letter stated that only 5

minutes is typically allocated for a doctor visit. It is because their schedules are based on financial considerations.

6. **High Costs and Affordability Issues:** Rising healthcare costs and medical expenses are a significant concern for many individuals. The high cost of prescriptions, medical procedures, and insurance premiums often lead to financial strain and difficulty accessing necessary care.

   Note: *The existing medical system is geared towards servicing rich people from a cost perspective, leaving the middle class and poor struggling to make ends meet.*

7. **Lack of Coordination and Continuity of Care:** Patients often report a fragmented healthcare system where coordination among different healthcare providers is insufficient, leading to duplicated tests, conflicting information, and inadequate follow-up care.

   Note: *When I was a child, a doctor might visit your home to check on you, especially in rural areas. The doctor would undoubtedly coordinate your care with other providers in those days. Not anymore. Today's medical system is highly fragmented, and unless you are your own advocate, you might get delivered the wrong* *meds, or god-forbid have the wrong body part operated on.*

8. **Insurance Denials and Limited Coverage:** Complaints about insurance companies denying coverage for necessary treatments, medications, or specialist referrals are commonplace. Limited coverage for specific procedures or medications can significantly impact patients' ability to receive adequate care.

It is hard to understand how our medical care has evolved to the point where actual health care is questionable, not for wealthy people but for the average person in the country on a limited budget. However, I want you to know it doesn't have to be this way for you and your family. Instead of paying excessive medical insurance costs, you can skip this approach to health and adopt an entirely different and more cost-effective approach. Let me explain another way of looking at health care. This one requires less fear and more self-care.

CHAPTER THREE
Assessing Health Risks

I was born in 1946 and grew up in the 50s and 60s. I joined the Navy in 1963, spending 7 1/2 years in Naval Missile Systems during the Vietnam War. I married young, and my wife and I had two daughters before I left the Navy. While in the service, I never gave a second thought to medical costs. The Navy provided our family's medical insurance and care. However, my wife and I experienced troubling and careless health care. After a miscarriage, the Naval Hospital nearly killed my wife by ignoring and not paying attention to her uterine hemorrhaging after a D&C. That was the first in a series of medical horror stories our family accumulated from using allopathic standardized medical services. It was not unusual for hospitals to pass off interns as regular doctors, albeit they were really "doctors in training."

As a youth, my poor parents taught me NOT to rush to doctors or hospitals. On one event, while spearfishing, my friend threw his spear into my left hand. Given the hooks on the spear, it wasn't easy to get the hook out of my hand. We waited for several days until the infection and inflammation were up to my elbow before going to see a doctor. Well, it all came out okay, and I survived the "let's see what happens" thinking for a few days before getting help. A friend of mine refers to this action as GBA or gets better anyway (without seeing a doctor.) In fact, a large percentage of injuries will get better on their own. It is because the body really wants to heal itself. The exceptions are acute injuries such as a broken bone or an infection moving up your arm.

My grandparents lived into their mid-90s. As far as I know, they never had any medical insurance. They just dealt with medical issues as they came up. The same thing happened with my parents, who also never had medical insurance. For most of my life, I also have not had any medical insurance. Today, at age 77, I do not have any medical insurance outside of the free Medicare Part A the government provides to those over 65. It gives some hospital coverage along with nursing home and hospice coverage. Still, without additional medical insurance, it is a prescription for bankruptcy.

I have no plans to get any additional coverage. In the 12 years I have had Medicare Part A, I have not used it once. If I have a medical issue, it is an out-of-pocket expense. Instead of paying hundreds of dollars each month for Medicare Parts B, C, and D, I have chosen to spend this level of money or more on products or activities that will improve my health. That would be on nutraceuticals, dentists, massages, etc. It means I spend money on improving my health each month and not on some medical insurance protection racket that provides me with virtually no genuine health care.

Health Risk Management

Think of your and your family's health care as a risk management task. Then, ask if your family is a moderate to heavy consumer of standardized medical (allopathic) doctor and hospital services. Now, in the context of risk management, you need to remember other forms of insurance you pay for also cover medical expenses. Suppose you are in an auto accident by yourself. Doesn't your automobile liability coverage also cover medical expenses if you are injured? Yes, it does. Likewise, suppose someone crashes into your car and causes the accident. In that case, their auto insurance will cover any costs over and above what your no-fault auto insurance medical will pay.

Are you prone to personal accidents, like falling down the stairs? Are you engaged in high-risk activities like climbing mountains or sky diving? Got kids? What about them? Do they play safely or engage in risky indoor or outdoor behavior? Does your family emphasize safe activities, or is safety a catch as catch can event.

What about your attitudes toward medical care? Do you run to the doctor at the first sign of a sniffle? Or can you take care of minor medical issues on your own? Do you understand almost all minor health issues will resolve on their own because the body wants to heal itself?

The financial reality is a fantastic amount of actual allopathic medical services can be paid for in cash before ever coming close to the premiums and deductibles being charged for medical health protection insurance.

The First Task

Therefore, your first task in any DIY health care plan is an assessment of your and your family's medical needs based on current behaviors and attitudes. This also includes assessing what costs you are willing to assume and take on yourself. This leads to at least four or more personal attitudes regarding medical insurance possibilities.

1) Your family consumes a lot of allopathic medical services and cannot afford to be without medical insurance. Even if you struggle with monthly costs and deductibles, it is too frightening to be without

medical insurance.

2) You're wealthy and not concerned about monthly costs and deductibles.

3) You're not a big consumer of medical services and tend to avoid doctors and hospitals. Still, your monthly costs and deductibles are manageable, and it's a peace of mind thing for you.

4) You tend to care for minor medical issues and think twice before rushing to a doctor. Your deductible is so high you know you'll have to pay out of pocket for thousands of dollars for any medical services. You might even have a health issue you are concerned about. However, you now find yourself weighing medical treatments against known deductible expenses. Your financial reality is your budget is being squeezed by excessive medical insurance costs, and you don't have any known options.

From my perspective, I don't believe in paying hundreds of dollars just for the privilege of obtaining a medical protection plan's peace of mind. It gets down to risk management, so instead, I have my own healthcare program. If I am going to spend money on health care, it should do something to actually improve my health. Yes, without an industry medical insurance plan, this means if I break an arm, I am out of pocket for getting it set and a cast put on it. However, I practice healthy living and manage the risks I take. I also understand that I can purchase a lot of standard medical services for the amount of monthly premiums the medical racketeers routinely demand.

Suppose your car is paid for, and you no longer have that $400-700 monthly car payment. Will you race out and get a new car, or will you save that money for the future? In the realm of cars, like all purchases, there are needs, wants, and desires. You might need a used Ford for transportation needs but want a new Honda or even desire a new Lexus SUV. The same concept applies to health care for you and your family. Your risk management task is to examine what you and your family really need to take care of medical concerns. This can differ significantly from what the medical industry wants you to pay or even what you desire. Like the prior analogy, you can afford to pay for a lot of maintenance on an old car and never come close to the cost of owning a new car.

One of the fundamental cost problems with our current medical system is the lack of individuality and the attempt to make one size fits all. Many years ago, in a business of mine, I was paying for our employee health care. Those costs included maternity care for my wife, who had her tubes tied three decades earlier. We did not need maternity coverage and had long ago stopped having children. When I complained, I was told it was state law, and I could not opt out of medical services I didn't need or want for this group insurance. It also required wigs for cancer patients who lost their hair during chemo and a host of other services we would like to opt out of if we could.

Today, in the Obamacare one-size-fits-all insurance scheme, the government mandates much medical coverage that many people do not need or want to pay for. One criticism is the requirement for approved health insurance plans to cover preventive services without cost-sharing, such as maternity, contraception, mammograms, prostrate, and cervical cancer screenings. In other words, federal and state governments mandate many medical procedures you may not need or want. The medical insurance industry is basically a collective medical insurance pool.

Suppose you are over 65, like me. In that case, you cannot purchase private insurance unless you first buy Medicare Part B from the government. Part B covers doctors, but good luck finding a doctor that accepts Medicare or Medicaid if you are unfortunate to be poor and on that government program. I suppose if I didn't have medicare shackles on me, I might lock into catastrophic medical coverage. Say something with a

$20,000 or higher deductible if I change my mind. It's unlikely, but it's still something I've thought about at various times. Theoretically, it should have a lower monthly cost, but that is not a given.

Another way of looking at risk management is to consider the choice between term-life insurance and whole-life insurance. If you are married and have young children, it's not hard to understand you need to protect your family in the case of your death. It's a financial reality that whole-term life insurance is out of the question for most families. That is why term-life insurance exists. It is an affordable insurance strategy for protecting a family if the primary wage earner dies. From age 25 to 75, I always carried $250-500k of term insurance to protect my family. If you are otherwise healthy, a term-life policy is an affordable insurance strategy.

Every 5-10 years, as I renewed or changed term policies, the life insurance company would put my body through an EKG, blood, and urine tests, along with an extensive questionnaire. It was always free of cost, constituting my periodic physicals. At age 65, I was rated for $500k coverage as a preferred customer by two insurance companies. It happened because all my life, I have sought to keep myself as healthy as possible and adopt good health habits. I stopped term insurance at age 74. I knew I would live beyond 75, and it was a waste of money at the time. After age 75, term life becomes exorbitantly expensive. It's an excellent risk management tool for young families.

You already determine your insurance needs and the level of the home, life, auto, umbrella, and other coverage. Often, however, no consideration is given to the dynamics of healthcare coverage for you and your family. The decision might be as simple as whatever health coverage your employer will provide or whatever you can afford.

Now, in this "Healing Self-Care DIY Plan," I am asking you to think outside the box of the traditional medical insurance protection racket. I am asking you to bet on the effects of living a healthy lifestyle and taking care of your own out-of-pocket medical expenses as they occur. It means not rushing to the doctor, hospital, or emergency room at the first sign of a sniffle. It means assessing whether the healthcare need is acute, minor, or a chronic issue you've been living with. It means doing your research and homework.

For me, I've decided to take care of myself to the best of my ability and to live with the consequences of my choices. It means I have decided to live like my father and grandfather did when it comes to medical concerns.

It doesn't mean I don't have any level of medical insurance at all. My house and auto insurance policies provide some medical insurance. My wife's HRA can offer some minor relief. The VA doctors and hospitals might be a fallback for some veterans, but not for me. I've ruled out any life-extending medical procedures like heart surgery, cancer treatments, etc.

I will give my body the best care possible during my earthly journey. When my time comes to exit the planet, I am ready. In other words, I will practice the same kind of medical care my parents and my paternal grandparents practiced. Take care of yourself, and don't rely on doctors. No matter what anyone asserts, only you can take care of your health, and like it or not, it is your responsibility.

It might surprise you that our modern concept of medical insurance didn't really start to take off until the late 1950s. Before then, people learned how to take care of themselves. Today, there are too many people not practicing enough self-care and instead are relying upon allopathic medical services to take care of their health. Isn't that why people rush to emergency services when they get a sniffle?

Now, I'll discuss what you might not know about allopathic medical services, doctors, and hospitals.

CHAPTER FOUR
Facts You Should Know

The Allopathic Medical System

You may not know that the following facts exist about our allopathic medical system. Doctors have spent twelve or more years obtaining a medical degree and the license to use their medical education. Given that reality, the first item on my list might shock you.

Suppose you've ever wondered about the unanimity of opinions in the medical industry. In that case, you should recognize that medical narratives about any disease and its treatments are now tightly controlled. Any attempt to advocate health solutions outside these controlled narratives can result in disciplinary action or even the loss of the right to practice medicine. Of course, it is against the law to practice medicine without a medical license.

Who would have thought that highly educated people could be so easily controlled by licensing organizations? The Covid-19 malaise revealed this "control" reality within the medical industry. I might add, with only a few exceptions for those brave enough to speak a different truth as they understood.

Facts You Need To Know

1) Highly educated medical doctors are controlled by the dictates of Big Pharma, along with the medical associations that license and regulate industry professionals.

2) Doctors are required to follow standardized medical procedures.

3) Doctors are trained by Big Pharma in the use of pharmaceuticals.

4) Doctors have little or no training in the use of vitamins and herbs for healing the body.

5) Doctors have little or no training in using nutrition or food in the body's healing.

6) Drugs prescribed by doctors only mask symptoms and do not address underlying health issues.

7) Doctors typically only offer you five minutes when you meet with them.

8) If you question your doctor's advice, they might get annoyed with you.

9) If you don't simply want a prescribed pill for your illness, you'll need to think outside the box of

standardized medical care.

10) There are emerging holistic doctors for health and healing. Consider alternative doctors who use nutrition, physical therapy, nutraceuticals, massage therapy, chiropractic treatments, and other modalities to enhance their standard medical practices. Naturopaths and functional doctors are two examples[1].

11) Allopathic standard medical practices are excellent at the treatment of acute health issues like broken bones, significant cuts, gunshot wounds, etc.

12) Allopathic standard medical practices are excellent at diagnostic testing of human body bones, tissues, blood, urine, stools, etc. There are a lot of diagnostic tools at the disposal of the medical industry.

13) Allopathic standard medical practices are mediocre or fail at treating chronic diseases like cancer, diabetes, or the many other metabolic diseases of the human body.

14) If you have a severe illness, you'll want to find an industry specialist in the illness who is not just a medical doctor.

15) It has been reported that 90% of oncologists would not take chemo themselves. Chemo destroys every living cell in your body. Having said that, new

medical treatments are being constantly developed, and the industry may have new options.

16) If you have cancer, the medical industry will not tell you that there exist many natural cures, such as high-dosage vitamin C treatments, oxygen treatment, etc. See "The Doctor's Death Diagnosis" book.

17) If you have a death diagnosis, the allopathic medical system will undoubtedly provide you with soothing care on your way off the planet.

18) There are many health issues similar to scurvy that are cured by food or vitamins. This fact is largely ignored by medical industry professionals, except for alternative doctor clinics.

19) It took over 100 years before medical doctors acknowledged that scurvy was a vitamin deficiency disease.

20) It took over 10 years before medical doctors would acknowledge that stomach ulcers were really the result of an H-pylori bacteria infection. This is despite the fact it was discovered by a medical doctor.

21) Medical doctors are trained to present themselves as the final authority on health issues and won't like discussing instructions.

22) Medical doctors, with the help of the PDR (physician's desk reference), will guess what drug to dispense to you. After all, with typically only 5 minutes per visit, they actually don't collect enough information for a more accurate health diagnosis.

23) With some minimal research, along with listening to your body, you can often make a more educated guess than the doctor about what your body is up against.

24) The human body wants to heal itself. It never amazes me when a body is healed. However, it does surprise me how much people can abuse their bodies and still stay alive. I have twice in my life seen a living skeleton walking. Which is to say someone walking with literal skin on their bones and very little muscle mass.

25) Trauma from our past and youth can affect our body's healing ability. Often, an emotional detox is required for the body to heal.

26) Our nutritional intake affects our body's ability to heal.

27) Our environment affects our body's ability to heal. If we are affected by toxic chemicals or environments, a chemical detox is required for the body to heal.

28) Healing has a spiritual construct as well. This construct deals with our belief system. If we believe we will die, then that belief will usually wind up in death regardless of the interventions used. Likewise, if we think we will be healed, we will usually get healed. See my blog and books for a detailed discussion.

29) Healing miracles happen, and I discuss several of them in my book *God And Healing*.

30) There is a list of "100 Healing Secrets And Tips" in *The Doctor's Death Diagnosis* book.

CHAPTER FIVE
1984 & Neo's Matrix

Welcome To 1984

I'm pretty confident that in George Orwell's imagination, he never saw the technology that now exists to control people. He saw the government controlling the people through their medical and news narratives. However, he didn't see the following technologies:

1) **The ability of software to modify photos on smartphones and other computer devices now exists.** The software can change seasons in photos: spring to winter, fall to spring, etc. It can remove people from a photo, add people to a photo, modify how a person looks in a photo, etc. If you look at a recent photo that you took, you can have a high degree of confidence it reflects the scene you shot. However, what about a photo someone you don't know shows you? Could you trust what you are looking at if the photo was not from a friend or family member?

2) **Photos are now being created or modified by AI (artificial intelligence).** AI is now capable of manufacturing fake photos that are photo-realistic. Over the past year, I saw some AI-created photos of President Trump being hauled away by the Police. Honestly, it would have been tough to guess if I didn't know AI created them.

3) **AI can now alter or create audio tracks in someone's voice.**

4) **AI can now alter or create videos in someone's image and voice.**

5) **News report narratives or propaganda can now be altered or created for the government by AI.**

6) **Search engine results like Google's are now highly filtered and controlled by powers intent on controlling people's thoughts.**

Welcome To Neo's Matrix

I remember when I saw the first Matrix movie. It stunned me for 1-2 weeks and kept me reflecting on my surroundings and environment. I had wound up in a Christian cult, which sounds like an oxymoron. Nothing was as it appeared to be. The congregation was totally being conned without anyone being the wiser. We were given narratives that were not true. To use a modern metaphor, we were all being gaslighted.

The pastor stole the church from its denomination and then from its congregation through fraudulent state articles and bylaw filings. It occurred behind everyone's back. It was the proverbial smiling to the congregation's face while simultaneously stabbing them in the back. He even paid for his daughter-in-law to divorce his son while he was busy serving in the Army. Then, he married his daughter-in-law and began raising his granddaughter as his own daughter. In 2023, his son started revealing what he knew. You can read the details[1] at www.james417.org.

There are so many matrix narratives in religion that it's almost incomprehensible. People believe all kinds of stuff that is not true. Having said that, religion is very fragmented and diverse. Unlike the medical industry, it does not have centralized control mechanisms.

The Medical Matrix

Today, medical narratives are very tightly controlled. The narratives cannot be 100% contained with all the bloggers and the internet. However, when all major news outlets and search engines are a part of the control apparatus, controlling 80-90% of what people believe and think about a given issue is what currently exists. Google, for example, filters out of search results any medical information deemed in opposition to the World Health Organization, CDC, FDA, and AMA's medical narratives.

Look no further than the narratives about the Covid-19 mRNA vaccine. Safe and effective? Some friends didn't even believe the vaccine was experimental. Yes, it was, and billions of people worldwide were unsuspectingly experimented on. Now, the results are coming in from around the world.

In recent news, it was reported by the CDC[2] that only 3.5% of the population in the USA have received the 2023 fall Covid-19 mRNA booster shot. Rasmussen said that 24%[3] of people claim to know someone who died or had severe complications from the mRNA vaccine shot.

Still, government gaslighting continues to convince everyone to get the latest Covid-19 booster shots. If the gaslighting is not working anymore, it is only due to word-of-mouth conversations about the disastrous Covid-19 experimental vaccines. According to the CDC, five percent of caregivers in ten states are now opting out[4] of childhood vaccinations for children. Non-vaccinated children have reached an all-time high, but why? Word-of-mouth? Many parents are starting to realize that childhood vaccinations[5] might be part of a medical matrix.

Perhaps the most interesting information in this

campaign is how people have now been led to believe that the common cold or flu season no longer exists. It is a fact that eight forms of the common cold are coronaviruses. However, there is little talk about getting the common cold or flu in the medical narratives. Instead, if you get the sniffles from the common cold, it could be Covid-19, and you can die from it unless you get the latest booster? Also, make sure you get an unreliable Covid-19 test?

Through relentless gaslighting, we've gone from making sure you wash your hands to avoid the flu and colds to "you're going to die from the sniffles unless you get a Covid-19 booster shot." The medical matrix has plans to implement mRNA vaccines for every conceivable illness and human sickness. Watch for more gaslighting on boosters you need.

There are good reasons to not trust the news nowadays. We do, in fact, live in a matrix. Maybe we are not locked up in a human body warehouse and used as batteries for a fictitious computerized world. However, life is not what it seems to be regarding medical options.

Alternative healing modalities are withheld by doctors who cannot reveal them without the risk of losing their medical licenses. Simple stuff like telling you high-dose IV vitamin-C treatments have been shown to cure cancer. Alternative healing strategies are not in their wheelhouse; if they know about them, they are forbidden to tell you anything not within standardized medical treatment modalities.

One disturbing and misleading healthcare strategy of the medical insurance industry is the promotion of medicare advantage plans. See this senate hearing on medicare advantage plans[6] YouTube video to fully understand the matrix illusion of medicare advantage plans. This would be considered Medicare Part C.

The government provides Medicare Part A free, which covers hospitals, nursing homes, and hospice care. They charge you for Part B, which covers doctors. Parts A and B only cover 80% of the bills, so seniors could face huge copayments. That is where Part C medicare advantage plans come into play. It is promoted and sold to seniors as the solution to cover all their expenses. Of course, it also doubles the monthly health care payments and limits seniors' options regarding health care services to the provider's network.

Regular Medicare has no network restrictions and requires no prior service approval. However, medicare advantage plans require prior approval for significant healthcare services. This senate hearing explains how medicare advantage plans restrict and deny services that would have otherwise been provided by regular Medicare Parts A and B. In other words, it's another healthcare matrix illusion that hides the underlying reality of healthcare services.

It's a particularly disgusting insurance scam because it's almost axiomatic that any bright senior might opt for a medicare advantage plan. Many of my retired relatives have such plans. However, if they really need serious health services, these plans will routinely deny or restrict otherwise available regular medicare services. Senate testimony states, "Medicare advantage plans are great until you really need them."

If you have a severe health issue, you will benefit by exploring alternative health and healing modalities. Two excellent online health resources you can search are:

- ✓ www.greenmedinfo.com - Sayer Ji has accumulated over 10,000 articles about alternative health and healing into a searchable database. I highly recommend subscribing to Green Med Info's email newsletter.

- ✓ www.healthmeans.com - Health Means has accumulated thousands of downloadable reports, talks, and other educational resources for every existing health condition. They also offer free online health seminars if you subscribe to their email newsletter. I highly recommend subscribing to Health Means' email newsletter.

Suppose you start your alternative health and healing

education at these two locations. In that case, I believe you will never regret the decision. I've spent years consuming their valuable alternative health and healing information. It's a great place to start getting informed on health and healing information hidden by the medical industry.

CHAPTER SIX
DIY Self-Care

Starting a DIY Self-Care Plan

If you've read this far, you are interested in DIY alternative health and healing for yourself and your family. At this point, I need to clarify what a DIY Self-Care Plan might entail. Any DIY Self-Care Plan has pros and cons. That is why the first step is assessing your and your family's health and making the best guesstimate of future health needs. By its nature, a DIY Plan has no guarantees that something catastrophic won't occur from a health perspective to someone in the family. However, it is essential to realize that modern medical insurance plans also do not offer any guarantees about future health conditions. Some degree of healthcare peace of mind directly results from good health habits and the daily consumption of essential supplements.

The only place I know that offers complete peace of mind on this earth exists only in the spiritual realm found within our minds. There is no absolute peace of mind regarding a health and healing strategy. Attempts to construct a medical insurance strategy that confers total peace of mind are impossible, even if an illusion of such peace is often presented. Financially wealthy families do have the ability to pay for whatever health care needs they may have. Perhaps that is the closest on the earth that people will ever get to a high degree of healthcare peace of mind. Middle-class and low-income people or families must focus on personal health habits, healthy behaviors, and the consumption of nutraceuticals to avoid healthcare worries.

Self-Care Attributes

What Can DIY Self-Care Mean?

It might mean that ...

1) You have decided to assume financial responsibility for some or all healthcare expenses for yourself and your family.

2) You do not have any doctor or hospital medical insurance.

3) You have decided to assume the costs of doctor visits.

4) You don't rush to the doctor over sniffles.

5) You attempt to deal with minor health issues without going to a doctor or emergency room.

6) You search for low-cost alternative health and healing strategies.

7) You reject routine allopathic medical testing, and instead, you get to know and listen to what your body is trying to tell you.

8) You might subscribe to a concierge medical clinic

offering a low monthly fee for all routine medical services if available nearby. Such clinics are now being established and will eventually spread across the United States. These clinics focus on keeping you healthy and are not just in the business of treating illnesses.

9) You think twice before accepting experimental mRNA vaccines without extensive human safety testing.

10) You recognize vaccines use aluminum as an adjuvant to cause immune systems to react faster and that it is toxic to the body.

11) You recognize vaccines may also contain thimerosal, a mercury-based preservative, which is also toxic to the body.

12) You understand that nutrition and nutraceuticals used in healing the body are not within the wheelhouse of most medical doctors.

13) You understand that health narratives are tightly controlled by forces in the medical industry and that doctors must follow standard medical practice dictates, or they could lose their license to practice. This revolves around prescribing drugs.

14) You understand that going to a clinic or regular doctor will usually result in a 5-minute consult and

the issuance of a drug from Big Pharma to consume.

15) You understand that doctors issue drugs, provide surgery, offer chemo and radiation treatments, and otherwise do not engage in treating the whole body. Allopathic medicine seeks only to reduce the symptoms. It does not seek to heal underlying health conditions that result in sickness.

16) You know that alternative doctors focus on nutrition and treating underlying conditions.

17) You take responsibility for your own health and healthcare expenses.

18) You understand that allopathic medical insurance may not cover alternative healing modalities designed to treat the whole body and not just reduce symptoms by using pharmaceuticals.

19) You understand a whole alternative industry of nutraceuticals exists that offers healing without the side effects that result from using pharmaceutical drugs.

20) You're willing to learn about alternative healing modalities and place them into practice for healing the body. This is because you know the body wants to heal itself if given the nutrients it needs.

21) You work to eliminate bad habits you know are

harming your health. These would include excessive alcohol consumption, smoking to any extent, including vaping, and any form of illegal drug use.

22) You work to eliminate prescription drug use when you find a replacement nutrient or nutraceutical solution from alternative doctors, clinics, or your research. You understand that some drugs require that the user titrate or be slowly weaned off for safety reasons. Going cold turkey off some drugs and even an alcohol addiction can have disastrous effects on the body that is used to them.

23) You do not worry about minor health issues that you can live with. Exploring allopathic medical cures for minor health issues can prove expensive and primarily unfruitful. If you currently have a minor or several minor health issues, focus your attention on finding alternative healing solutions.

24) There are alternative health solutions for diabetes, cancer, heart, and many other health issues that humans experience. These are not medical issues per se but should be considered the body's health and healing needs.

25) You understand the GBA[1] concept in that regardless of treatment or no treatment, the body will get better anyway (GBA).

Now, let's consider what a DIY basic Self-Care might look like from my perspective. After that, we'll view some advanced additions to the basic self-care DIY plan.

Basic DIY Self-Care

1) You first assessed the family's health and the degree of medical financial risk-taking you are comfortable with.

2) You then reviewed what a DIY Self-Care plan might entail and acknowledged the reality of those attributes.

3) You understand that cash outlays could occur every month for medical expenses, even though you may not be paying a monthly healthcare premium for medical insurance.

4) You feel spending your limited cash resources on health care needs is better than only paying for medical insurance.

5) DIY Self-Care plans can pay for your and your family's vitamins and other nutritional support needs. It can pay for alternative healing modalities like massage, chiropractic care, etc. These are health and healing expenses for the body that medical insurance usually does not cover. In this manner, your medical cash outlays are working to improve your and your family's health. You are

paying to enhance health and healing and not just for some insurance protection.

Note: This doesn't mean your medical or health expenditures will be tax deductible. Tip: See your tax accountant and ask whether setting up a single-employee C-corporation or other business structure might benefit from the tax deductibility of your current medical expenses.

A Basic Self-Care Plan

1) <u>Move Your Body</u>: Human bodies are meant to move. That means there should be regular movements like walking, stretching, light exercise, routine chores, other movements, etc.

2) <u>The Body Has A Fascia Layer</u>: Around every muscle, organ, and bone is a layer of tissue called the fascia[1]. Consider it a layer of lubricant around body parts that allows body parts and muscles to move quickly, etc. ***Caution:*** *If you do not move your body, fascia can dry up, and body parts that aren't being moved enough may get very stiff and rigid to move. See the YouTube video link in the notes.*

3) <u>Hydrate Your Body</u>: The human body is 60%

water[2]. You must keep yourself hydrated, as many health issues can be traced directly to dehydration. It's easy to diagnose your hydration level by testing the skin on the top of your hands or looking at the color of your urine. You can pinch the skin on the top of your hand and observe how fast it will return to normal. Urine that is dark in color indicates your body is dehydrated. Drink when you are thirsty and try to consume 40-50% of your body weight in ounces of water as a hydration target. For example, 120 pounds would target 48-60 ounces[3] of water daily. ***Caution: Don't over-consume water, as it can be dangerous.***

4) <u>Consume A Daily Multivitamin</u>: Consuming a multivitamin is essential to any DIY Self-Care Plan. For men[4] and women[5], I would recommend the Synergy Multivitamins, found online at Vitacost.com[6]. For men, there are six pills/day, and for women, eight pills/day. Choose the multivitamin without iron, as it's doubtful you need additional iron unless you are under a doctor's care for low iron issues. Work slowly up to the total pills/day if you've never taken a quality multivitamin before. The body often needs a few weeks to fully adapt to a quality nutraceutical regimen you are not used to. That applies to all

new nutrients you might add to your diet.

5) <u>Supplement With Magnesium</u>: Most bodies lack sufficient magnesium, which supports over 300 body functions. Take 200 mg of magnesium in the morning and 200 mg an hour before bed. There are many different types of magnesium. I recommend magnesium glycinate[7]. Avoid magnesium oxide because it has poor absorption. Odds are your multivitamin will not have sufficient magnesium to satisfy body needs.

6) <u>Supplement With Vitamin C</u>[8]: Most bodies will benefit from taking 2,000 to 5,000 mg daily. Split your dosage throughout the day to maximize its efficiency.

7) <u>Supplement Zinc With Quercetin</u>: According to alternative doctors, you should get 60-200 mg of zinc daily. Take it with quercetin to maximize the healing impact of zinc.

8) <u>Supplement With D3</u>: Try to get 5,000 to 10,000 IU units of Vitamin D3 into your body daily to maximize health. Take it with magnesium for maximum effectiveness.

9) <u>Supplement With Essential Fatty Acids</u> (EFAs): These are fish oils[9] that eliminate inflammation in the body, lubricate joints, feed the brain, and do

much more in terms of healing.

10) <u>Supplement With Probiotics</u>: Much healing comes directly from the gut's microbiome. Feed your microbiome's good bacteria[10] if you want to live a healthy life. Sauerkraut, kimchi, yogurt, etc., also feeds your microbiome.

That is what I see as a minimal basic health plan. It won't negate lousy health habits, but it will improve your health despite bad habits. As an adult, I believe this is a good health plan. It will help keep you out of doctor's offices and hospitals. Kids should be on a daily multivitamin suited for kids and other nutrients. It would be best if you did some research to determine what you and your family need for their own DIY Self-Care plan.

Many low-cost nutrients you can find at discount and variety stores contain polypropylene glycol. You might recognize this as anti-freeze. It is toxic to the body and used primarily to keep nutrients from freezing. You should skip all products that use this ingredient as it is unhealthy.

Consider some advanced nutrients you can use or add to the above basic plan.

DIY Basic Plan Additions

If you need healing or want to further enhance your body's health and healing, consider adding one of the following nutrients to your basic DIY plan.

- Borage Oil[1] - I use this product as part of my anti-inflammation protocol. It contains Gamma Linolenic[2] Acid (GLA), which, according to one author, helps arthritis sufferers. It enhances healing within the body.

- H2 Molecular Hydrogen[3] - A small pill that dissolves in water and provides a hydrogen-enhanced drink. You dissolve the pill in 12-16 ounces of water and then drink it down immediately. There are many benefits of H2-enhanced water. It enhances healing within the body.

- Turmeric[4] - Enhances healing within the body.

Many other nutrients can assist healing in your body. However, the above three nutrients are near the top of my list. Many other nutrients are known to improve the longevity of your life, such as niacinamide[5] and astragalus[6].

What Would Ed Do?

I have provided valuable healthcare resources in this short "Healing Self-Care Primer." The first step in your DIY Plan is to assess the health risks you or your family can financially or emotionally assume. This health risk assessment forms the foundation of your health and healing strategy. From it will come monthly cash outlays to support the health and healing DIY plan you adopt.

Your second step is to research significant health issues you or your family have in search of alternative and low-cost healing strategies. I have presented some easy ways to analyze low-cost and alternative healing strategies. However, searching for alternative health and healing cures can get complicated.

In this regard, I have a strategy to help you with your DIY self-care. After doing your research, if you come up empty-handed, you can go to one of three feedback forms and contact me. These contact forms are at the following websites:

1)   www.edwardgpalmer.com/contact.html

2)   www.godandhealing.org/contact.html

3)   www.thedoctorsdeathdiagnosis.com/contact.html

Using one of these three forms, you can tell me your situation and ask me what I would do if I had (name the health issue).

I might contact you for additional information, respond with an answer of what I would do, or write a blog about my approach. When I do respond, it should NOT be considered medical advice. It would only be educational advice from my personal perspective. It would represent things I would do in that particular health situation.

I may already have an answer as to what I would do if I were in your shoes. If not, my extensive health library and computer health files may have an answer I can share. It is my earnest desire to help people understand that we do have options when it comes to medical care.

What Is Your Body Telling You?

Health issues should be considered something your body is telling you that it needs. It doesn't mean automatically rushing to a doctor, hospital, or emergency room for expensive standard medical services. Every DIY self-care strategy acknowledges that options, choices, and tradeoffs come with each health issue. DIY options and choices are inexpensive, and allopathic medical options and choices are expensive. The trigger for choosing an allopathic medical option or choice should be whether or not you are dealing with an acute medical crisis. Non-acute health issues can usually be dealt with using DIY self-care.

May God bless you and your family with health throughout your earthly journey. I hope this DIY Primer has given you a different perspective on health care.

Edward G. Palmer, Author

CHAPTER SEVEN
DIY Self-Care Resources

Take the time to research alternative health and healing strategies. You will learn that a massive amount of information is already at your fingertips. How do you know what advice is valid and what advice you should ignore? Since researching health care nuggets for over 50 years, I have established some basic information strategies that work for me.

Seven Alternative Health Information Rules:

1) If I hear something I know is a blatant lie or is uninformed from my perspective, I will block that expert or website. Information changes in many fields now at a rapid pace. Therefore, before you block a resource, you owe it to yourself to consider whether or not what you are exposed to is new information or something and someone to ignore when it comes to medical advice.

2) You've taken action on some advice and have

found out from personal experience that it was good advice. Add that expert or website to your allow list of trusted health advisors.

3) You've discovered that at least two or more potential health advisors offer the same advice. For example, Vitamin C in large doses applied via an IV into a vein can cure cancer. Oxygen therapy can cure cancer, etc. When you hear the same advice from multiple alternative health and healing sources, you should pay attention and do some research. Such information might be something you can personally use.

4) Suppose you are researching health issues on any allopathic medical site. In that case, you need to realize that alternative healing options are either not presented or steeply discounted as dangerous, not valid, or even medical quackery. Consider laetrile or Vitamin B17 in treating cancer, which was discovered in the 1950s by G. Edward Griffen[1]. You can also consider Olive Leaf Extract and Celery Seed Extract for the natural elimination of high blood pressure problems.

5) You can use ChatGPT and other A.I.s to research health issues but be aware that they are being programmed with allopathic medical treatments. While it won't provide alternative health

Healing Self-Care: A DIY Primer

information, it should give you a better understanding of standard medical treatment modalities. Same thing is true with Google's search engine. Use www.duckduckgo.com if you are in a generalized health information search.

6) You can use YouTube.com to learn standard medical and alternative health advice. See Doctor Eric Berg's health channel. He has extensive health information dealing with a lot of issues the body is confronted with such as bladder[2], knee, neck, and back pain, etc. See also the *motivationaldoc* channel of Doctor Alan Mandell. I have found practical DIY health solutions on these channels. I learned a neck[3] muscle massage strategy from Mandell that has greatly relieved neck pain. He also teaches a bent-over stretch that greatly relieves mid[4]-back[5] pain.

7) There are countless alternative health books, eBooks, pdfs, and health seminars that will cost you money. Don't be afraid to spend a few bucks to save perhaps hundreds of bucks by using DIY strategies first before seeking allopathic medical services.

On my author's website[6], I have a blog focused primarily on health and healing issues. You can also access the two health and healing books I've written, *God And Healing* and *The Doctor's Death Diagnosis*.

God And Healing is a book I wrote to provide the spiritual side of healing that I believe God has provided us with in Scripture. Again, the body wants to heal itself. However, we must get out of our own way and understand that the spiritual side of healing our bodies is essential.

On page 15-16, you will find a list of Scriptures regarding healing our body to reflect on.

On pages 17-52, you find discussions about stress and worry and a known strategy for dealing with these issues.

On pages 53-54, you will find a list of 37 items affecting your body's healing ability.

On page 67 there is a discussion of how habits affect the body.

On page 69, you'll find a list of healing verses to pray over sick friends or family members. You can also use them on your own body.

This small book of only 124 pages discusses how faith or lack of faith can impact your body's ability to heal itself. It concludes with my divine healing formula that I believe will work for people of all faiths regardless of religion.

The Doctor's Death Diagnosis is a book I wrote to explain DIY Self-Care and alternative healing strategies in more detail than what is possible in this short DIY Self-Care Primer.

On page 238, you'll find a list of twelve (12) alternative doctors I trust.

On pages 239-240, you'll find a list of forty (40) alternative health websites I trust.

On page 237, you'll find a list of seventeen (17) health signs that everyone should be concerned about.

On pages 229-236, you'll find a list of sixty-two (62) nutraceutical secrets I've learned over the years.

On pages 217-228, you'll find a list of one hundred (100) healing secrets and tips I've learned from 50+ years of life experiences in DIY Self-Care.

Since digital versions of these health and healing books are available for only $2.99, it is a low cost way of getting educated in DIY self-care methodologies. I hope these writings will take some of the financial and other burdens off your back regarding your and your family's health care. Do take some time to write me if you found my writings were of help to you.

Free Cancer Resource

After my first wife died of pancreatic cancer, I wrote a short healing eBook called *God's Healing And Cancer Protocols*. It summarizes the cancer-healing information I found at that time. It is available as a $7.95 pdf eBook. It is also available free to read within a web browser. It is located on my cancer information website[7]. Click on the legacy website link to read this cancer information free. You will find a browser link at the bottom of the legacy webpage. Suppose you need a starting point for how to deal with a cancer diagnosis using alternative healing strategies. In that case, this is the place to start.

Covid-19 Spike Protein Resource

Injury reports[8] are coming out about bodily damage caused by the spike proteins from the mRNA Covid-19 vaccines. As a result, many people are concerned with how they can eliminate the spike proteins in their bodies. Doctor Peter McCullough, a cardiologist, and other alternative doctors have formed The Wellness Company[9]. They have created a nutraceutical product focused on Nattokinase to eliminate the spike proteins in the body. They have also created an emergency medical kit [10]to get you ready for the next crisis should one occur. This group is focused on medical freedom and is another go-to alternative healing website.

A Self-Care Library

There are a massive amount of healing self-care and alternative healing strategy books available. Here are three healing self-care book resources to start or add to your healthcare library. I highly recommend all three books as valuable self-care health resources.

1) **Prescription for Nutritional Healing**[11], Sixth Edition. A Practical A-to-Z Reference to Drug-Free Remedies Using Vitamins, Minerals, Herbs & Food Supplements. Phyllis A. Balch, CNC (See notes).

2) **The Lost Book Of Herbal Remedies**[12]: The Healing Power of Plant Medicine. Nicole Apelian, Ph.D & Claude Davis. (See notes).

3) **Doctor Yourself: Natural Healing That Works**[13], Second Edition, Andrew W. Saul, Ph.D. (See notes).

Notes

Introducing Healing Self-Care Author

1. You'll find "God And Healing" at http://www.godandhealing.org. There are five versions of the book available including a $2.99 ePub and Kindle edition.
2. You'll find "The Doctor's Death Diagnosis" at http://www.thedoctorsdeathdiagnosis.com. There are five versions of the book available including a $2.99 ePub and Kindle edition.

Facts You Should Know

1. A more detailed discussion of the fractured medical industry and treatment options can be found in the book "The Doctor's Death Diagnosis."

1984 & Neo's Matrix

1. http://www.james417.org is where you can read about the story of Solid Rock Church in Elk River MN, and Pastor William Neal Matthews.
2. https://www.nytimes.com/2023/10/27/health/covid-vaccination-rates.html
3. https://www.rasmussenreports.com/public_content/politics/public_surveys/killer_jab_24_say_someone_they_know_died_from_covid_19_vaccine
4. https://www.aol.com/news/parents-opting-routine-childhood-vaccines-012705047.html
5. https://vaccines.news
6. Senate's medicare advantage plan expose is at https://www.youtube.com/watch?v=4PvqksIEN-M

Self-Care Attributes

1. Thanks to my friend Rick for expressing this GBA (gets better anyway) medical concept to me. It parallels the idea that colds get better in 7-10 days regardless of what you do. It's because the body wants to heal itself.

Basic DIY Self-Care

1. See video at https://www.youtube.com/watch?v=raCBeQ-gXfs&list=PLp8P2iUYSVWIlYHeVNSRE84xTxp_jwms0&index=4
2. https://www.medicalnewstoday.com/articles/what-percentage-of-the-human-body-is-water
3. This is my personal estimate of the water intake to keep your body hydrated.
4. https://www.vitacost.com/vitacost-synergy-mens-multivitamin-180-capsules
5. https://www.vitacost.com/vitacost-synergy-womens-multivitamin
6. Vitacost is where I buy almost all of my vitamins, herbs, and nutraceuticals. I have used them for years and usually find the best prices and service.
7. https://www.vitacost.com/kal-magnesium-glycinate-350
8. https://www.vitacost.com/vitacost-synergy-advan-c-1-000-mg-per-serving-with-quercetin-bioflavonoids?ta=vitamin+c&t=vitamin+c
9. https://www.vitacost.com/vitacost-synergy-mega-efa-1200-mg-omega-3-epa-dha-per-serving?ta=mega+efa&t=mega+efa
10. https://bluebiology.com/products/bluebiotics-ultimate-care - This is my choice for probiotics to feed our microbiome.

DIY Basic Plan Additions

1. https://www.vitacost.com/now-borage-oil?ta=borage+oil&t=borage+oil
2. You can start your study of GLA here - https://www.nordic.com/healthy-science/health-benefits-of-gla/
3. https://www.mercolamarket.com/category/1761/1/h2-molecular-hydrogen

4. https://www.vitacost.com/vitacost-root2-turmeric-ext-curcumin-c3-complex-with-bioperine
5. Number one nutrient for healing bad knees according to the vitamin man, Dr. Andrew Saul. See this video on YouTube - https://www.youtube.com/watch?v=iPZ4UyOl7Ps
6. Considered the number one nutrient to extend telameres in the body. This lengthens the amount of cellular division possible and can result in growing younger as you age according to one longevity expert.

DIY Self-Care Resources

1. G. Edward Griffin postulates in his video "World Without Cancer - The Story of Vitamin B17" documentary that cancer is another nutrient deficiency in the body. You can view his documentary on YouTube at https://www.youtube.com/watch?v=tPADSv3XAv0
2. See https://www.youtube.com/watch?v=ElKTOnm2kEw and other health videos from Dr. Eric Berg's extensive DIY YouTube channel.
3. See https://www.youtube.com/watch?v=fe0yBAxQYE4 and other neck muscle videos to relieve neck pain. These are simple body hacks that do not cost you any money but only a small amount of time for some instant pain relief.
4. See https://www.youtube.com/shorts/S8aGUBakgMs. This is the stretch that greatly relieved my mid back pain. I practice this stretch a few times every week to keep pain free in my mid-back.
5. See https://www.youtube.com/watch?v=GxWgDQCuNTs and other back pain videos for simple body hacks to relieve pain. This stretch will also relieve hamstring pain under the thigh and a slight variation will relieve IT band pain on the outside of the knees.
6. http://www.edwardgpalmer.com/blog.html
7. http://www.informcentral.org
8. https://www.zerohedge.com/news/2023-11-06/covid-propaganda-roundup-unreal-poll-results-jab-death-toll-sciencetm-concedes
9. You can find them online at https://www.twc.health.
10. https://thelibertydaily.com/before-next-crisis-hits-prepare-medical-emergency-kit/
11. https://www.amazon.com/Prescription-Nutritional-Healing-Sixth-Supplements/dp/0593330587/ref=sr_1_1?

crid=6FLESIXGGI4Y&keywords=prescription+for+nutritional+heali
ng&qid=1699312982&sprefix=prescript%2Caps%2C328&sr=8-1

12. https://www.amazon.com/Lost-Book-Remedies-Claude-Davis/dp/
     1732557101/ref=sr_1_1?
     crid=2JT1FPU4YZSD4&keywords=the+lost+book+of+herbal+remedi
     es+by+nicole+apelian&qid=1699313278&sprefix=the+lost+book+
     %2Caps%2C126&sr=8-1

13. https://www.amazon.com/Doctor-Yourself-Natural-Healing-
     Works/dp/1591203104/ref=sr_1_1?
     crid=UUOSFLFAC9ED&keywords=doctor+yourself+andrew+saul&
     qid=1699313472&sprefix=doctor+your%2Caps%2C124&sr=8-1

About The Author

Edward G. Palmer has studied alternative health and healing issues for over 50 years. He considers himself a "Healing Self-Care" expert and is sought after for his alternative healing and nutraceutical strategies.

He took his first comprehensive multivitamin at the age of 25 in 1971. Already in excellent health and with plenty of energy, Ed was surprised at how this multivitamin enhanced his health and vitality in a way he could not deny. That early life experience began a lifelong effort to use vitamins and other nutraceuticals, such as herbs, to enhance his health.

Ed quickly concluded that he could not bet his health on being able to eat well. Instead, Ed decided he would eat the healthiest he could but would bet his overall health and longevity on nutraceuticals.

As a child, Ed's parents taught him by their own example to care for himself and not rely on doctors for his health and healing. The biggest lesson learned early in life was that we are all personally responsible for our own health.

Author & Publisher

Author Information

Edward G. Palmer

13570 Grove Drive #361

Maple Grove MN 55311

http://www.edwardgpalmer.com

Publisher Information

JVED Publishing

13570 Grove Drive #361

Maple Grove MN 55311

http://www.jvedpublishing.org

Related Self-Care Health Books

God And Healing: A Bible Perspective

This 6 x 9" book discusses what the Bible says about Divine healing. Will God always heal as a result of prayer? It is available in Print, PDF, and $2.99 eBook editions. Details at http://www.godandhealing.org

The Doctor's Death Diagnosis

This 6 x 9" book discusses alternative healing strategies to allopathic medicine. It has a list of "100 Healing Secrets & Tips." It is based on the author's 50-year experience using alternative health strategies. It is available in softcover Print, hardcover Print, low-cost PDFs, and $2.99 eBooks. Details are found at http://www.thedoctorsdeathdiagnosis.com.

Other Books & Writings

Several other books are available and several free to read writings of the author. You can find them at the publisher's website. The free writings are found towards the bottom of the publisher's home page. http://www.jvedpublishing.org.